THE FOOD GROUPS FOR KIDS

BY BOLD HEARTS PUBLISHING

&BRYANT BILLUE

BASED ON THE
DIETARY GUIDELINES FOR AMERICANS

THERE ARE 5 FOOD GROUPS

1. **VEGETABLES**
2. **FRUIT**
3. **PROTEIN**
4. **GRAINS**
5. **DAIRY**

EACH GROUPS INCLUDES FOOD THAT YOU EAT EVERYDAY.

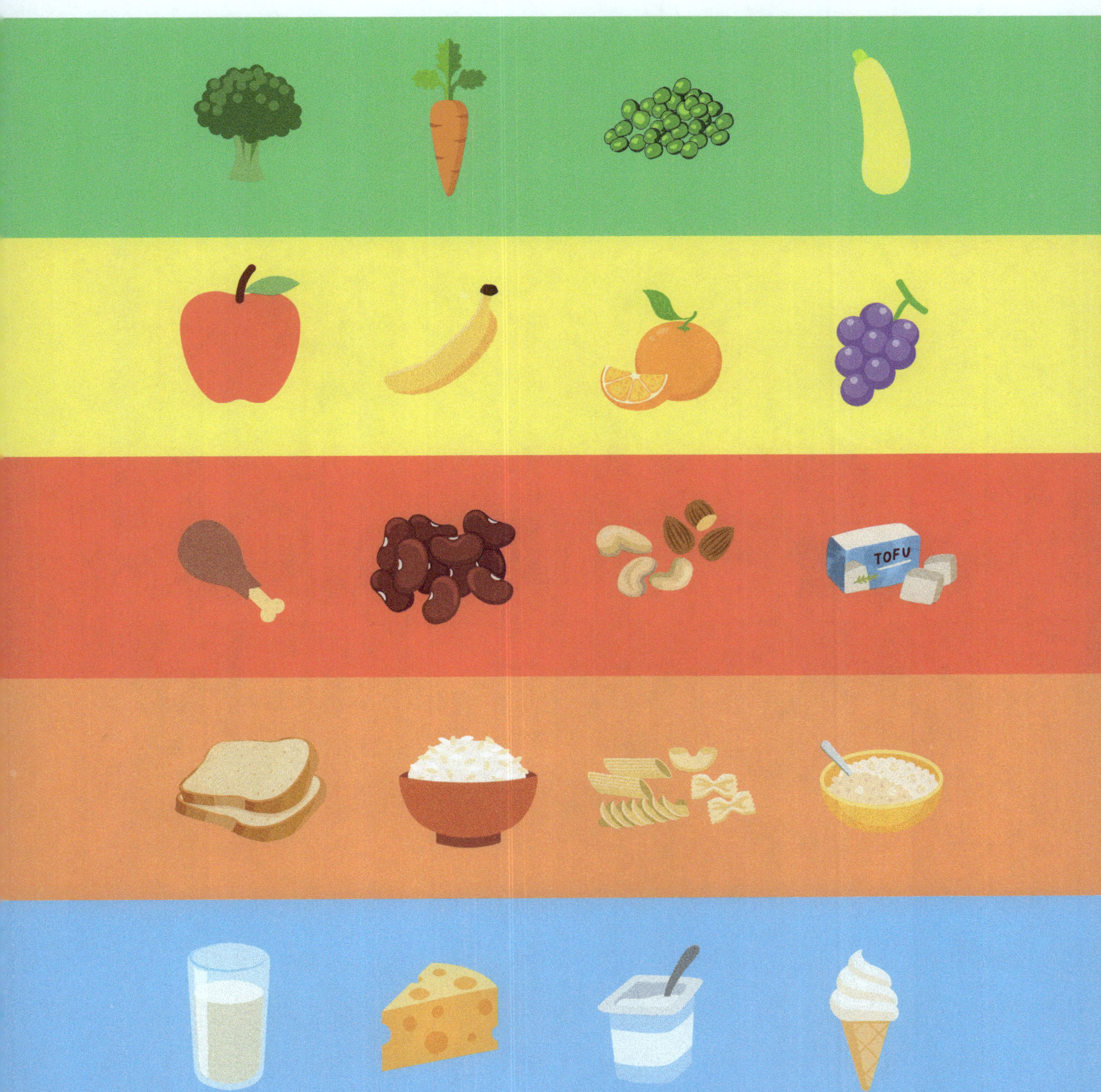

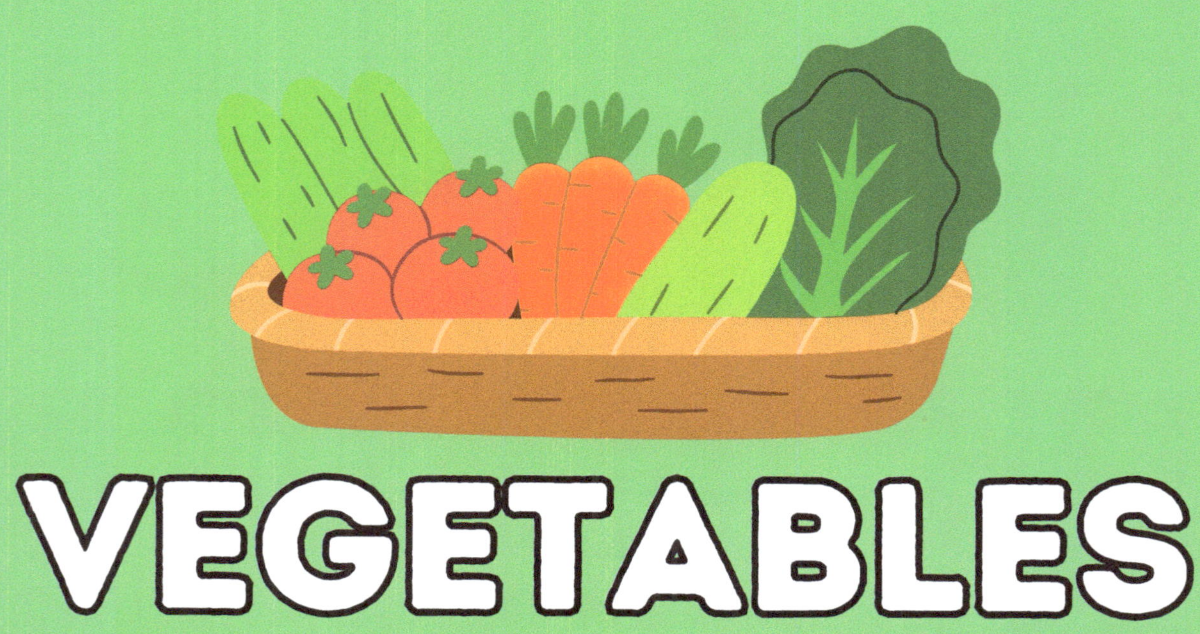

VEGETABLES

THESE FOODS
ARE IMPORTANT
FOR BODY FUNCTIONS
LIKE VISION AND HEALING.

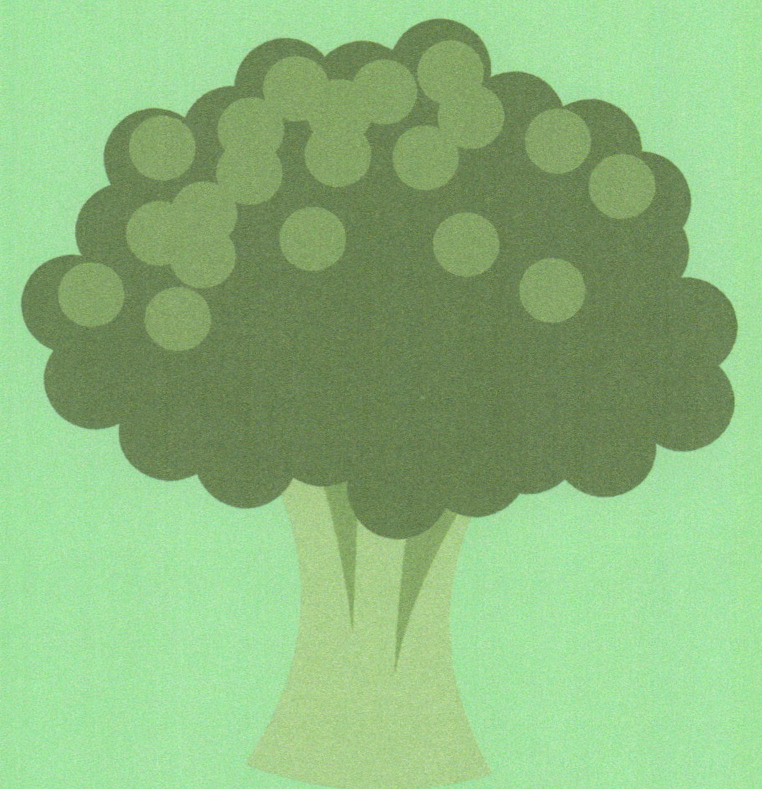

BROCCOLI

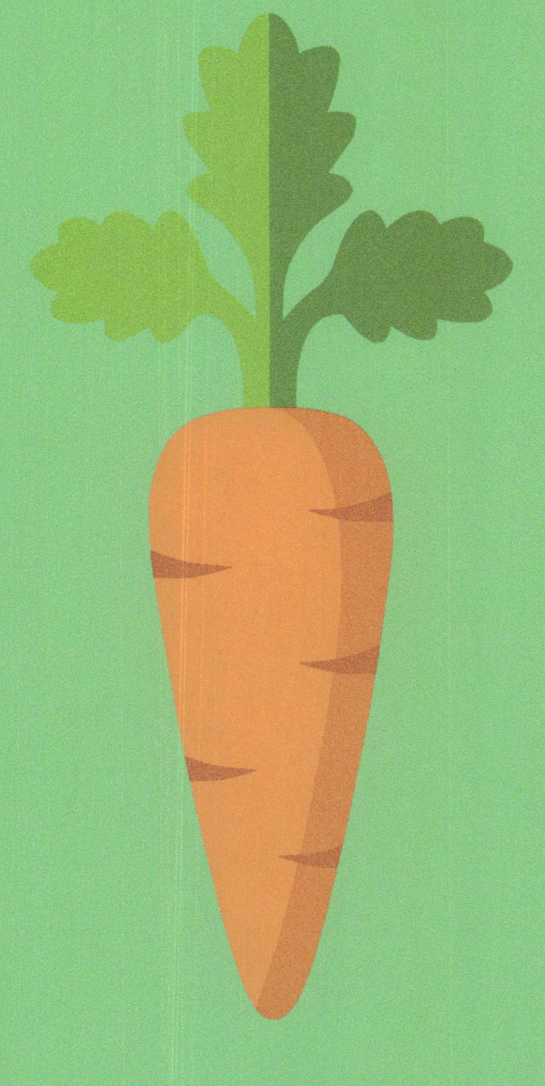

CARROT

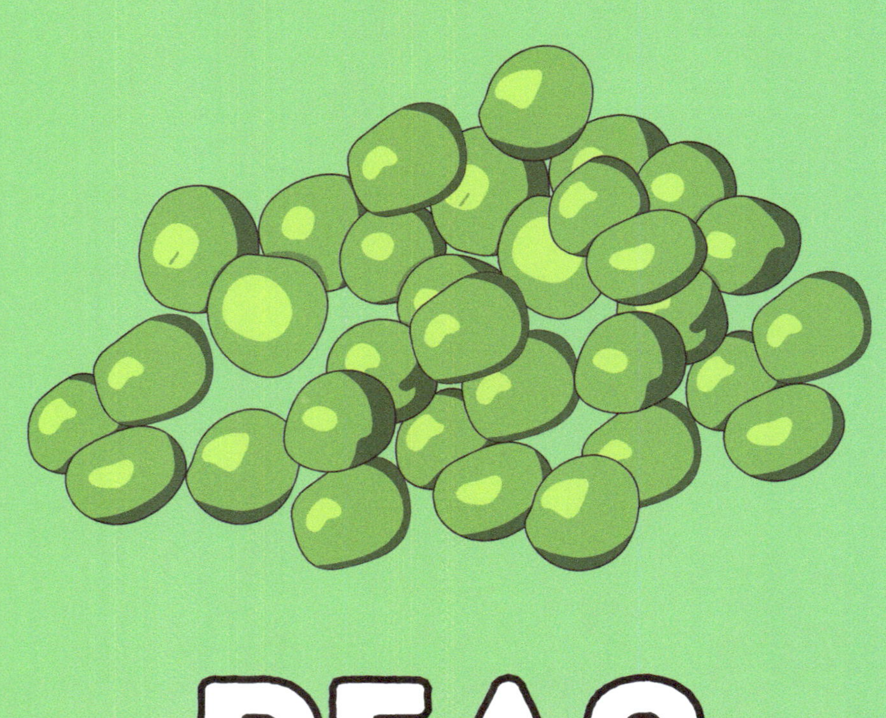

PEAS

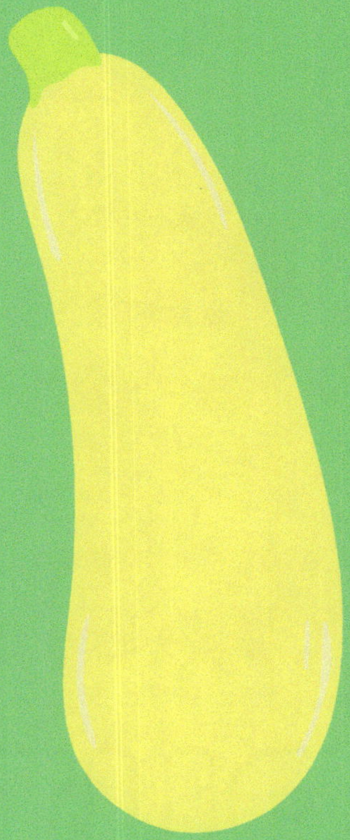

SQUASH

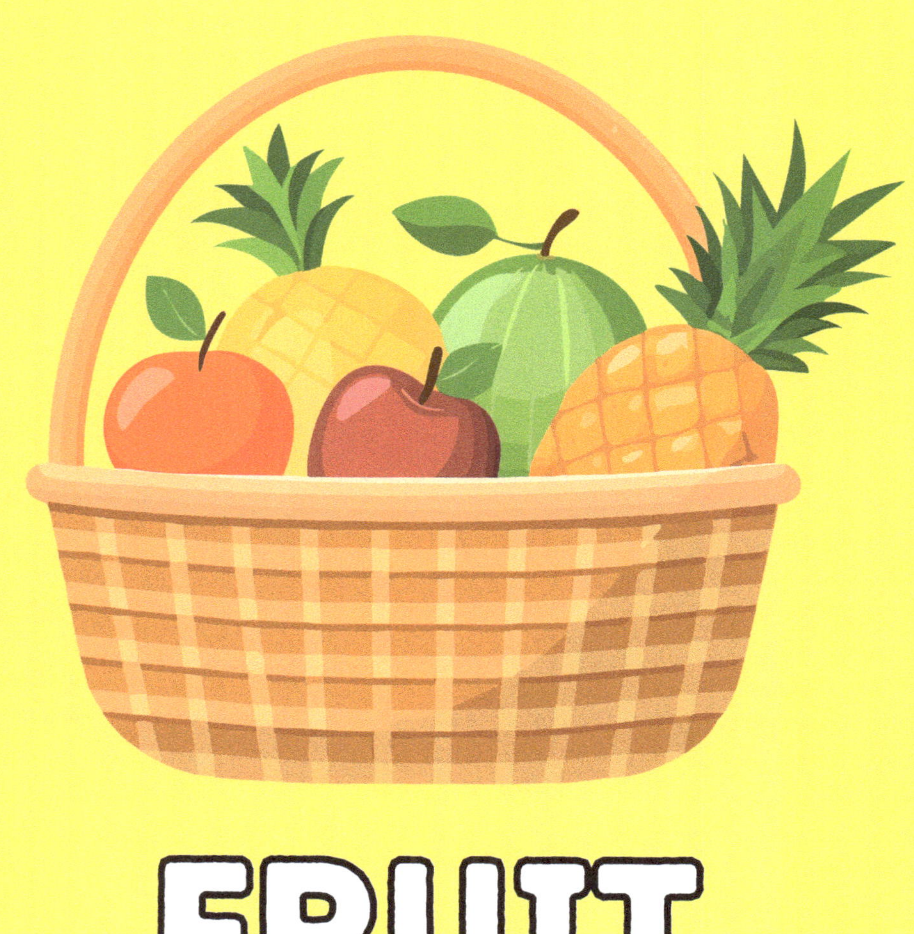

FRUIT

THESE FOODS ARE FULL OF VITAMINS THAT PREVENT YOU FROM BECOMING SICK!

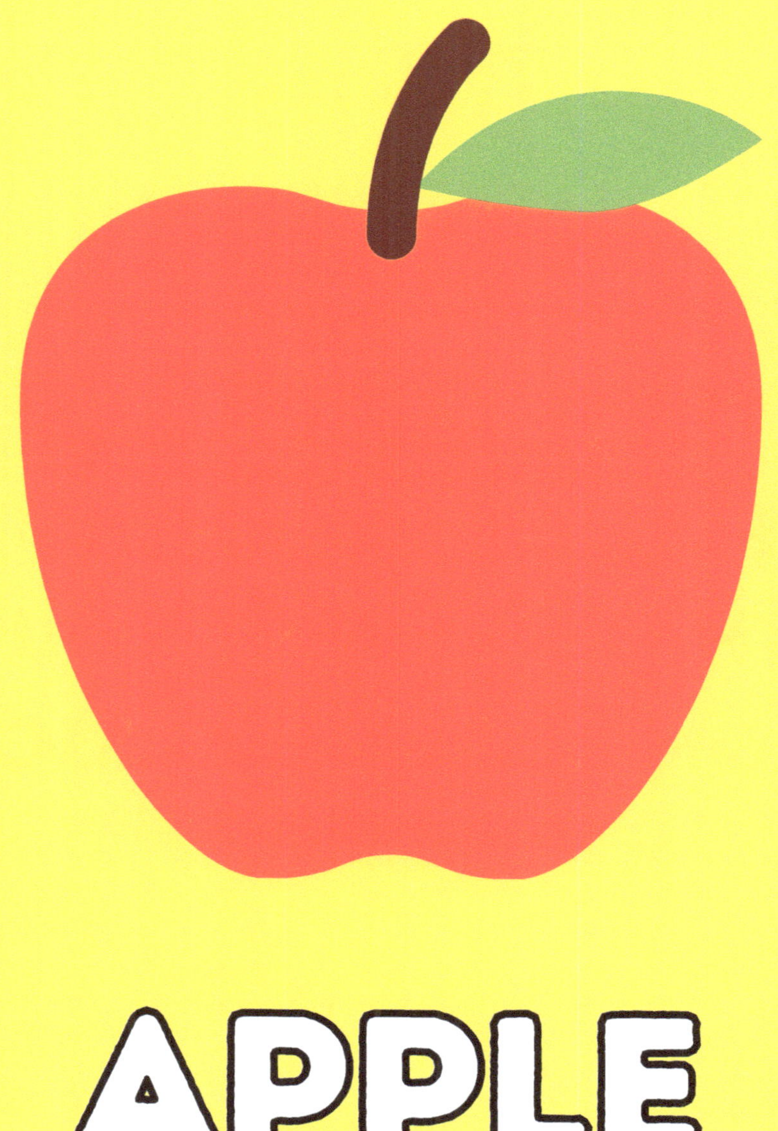

APPLE

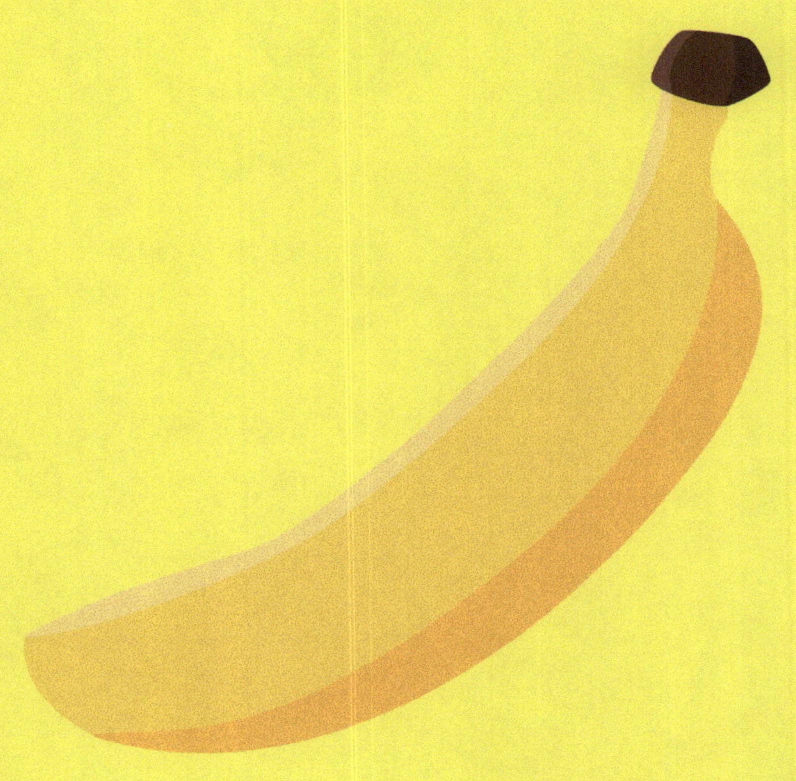

BANANNA

ORANGE

GRAPES

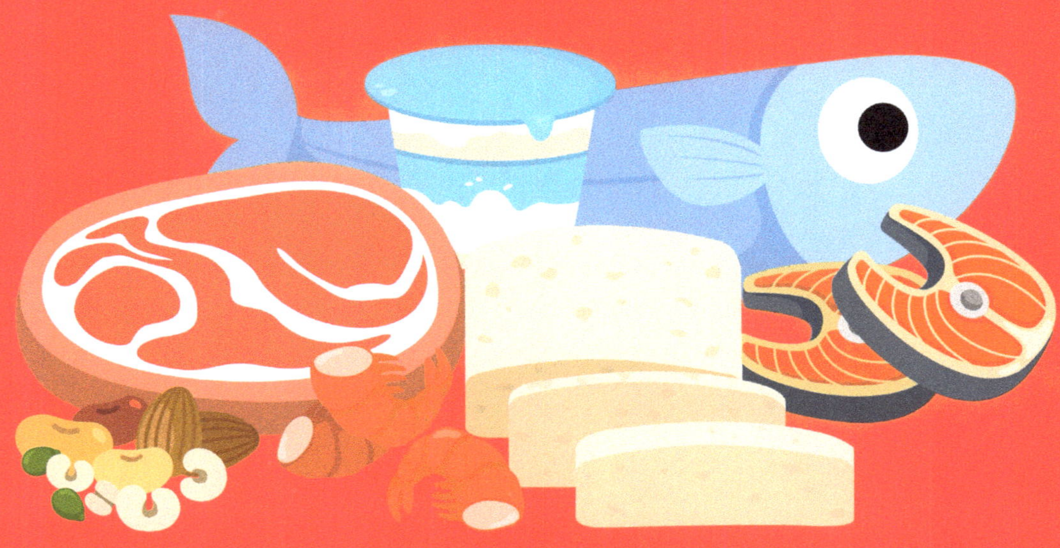

PROTEIN

THESE FOODS MAKE
OUR MUSCLES STRONG!

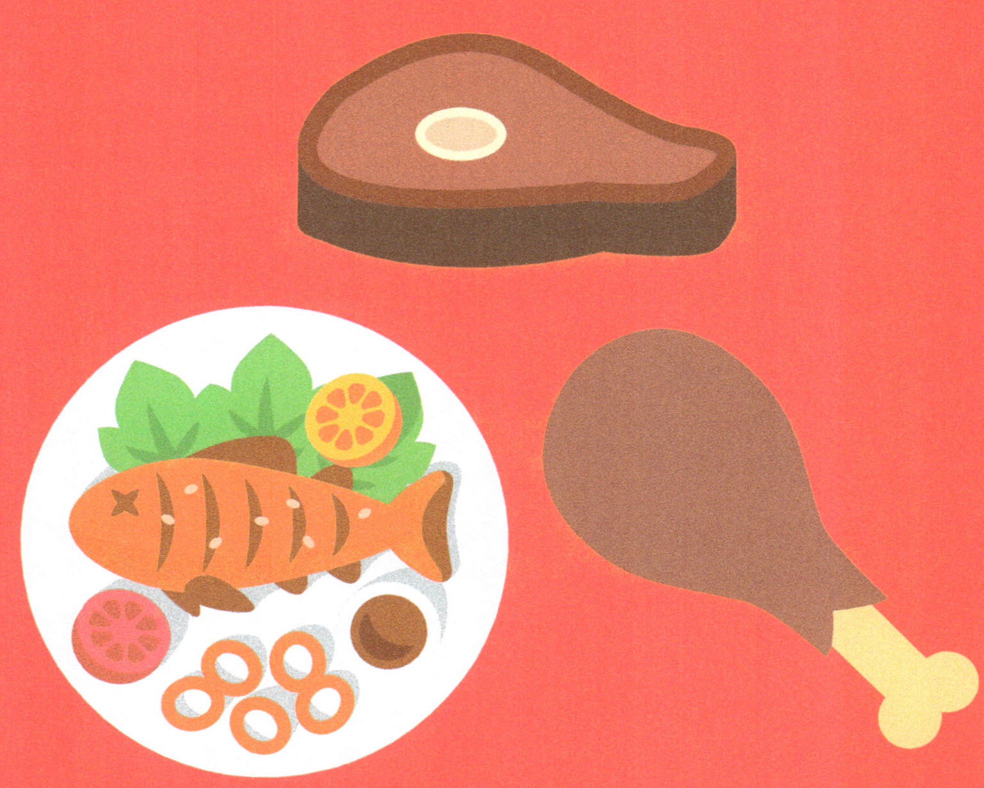

MEAT

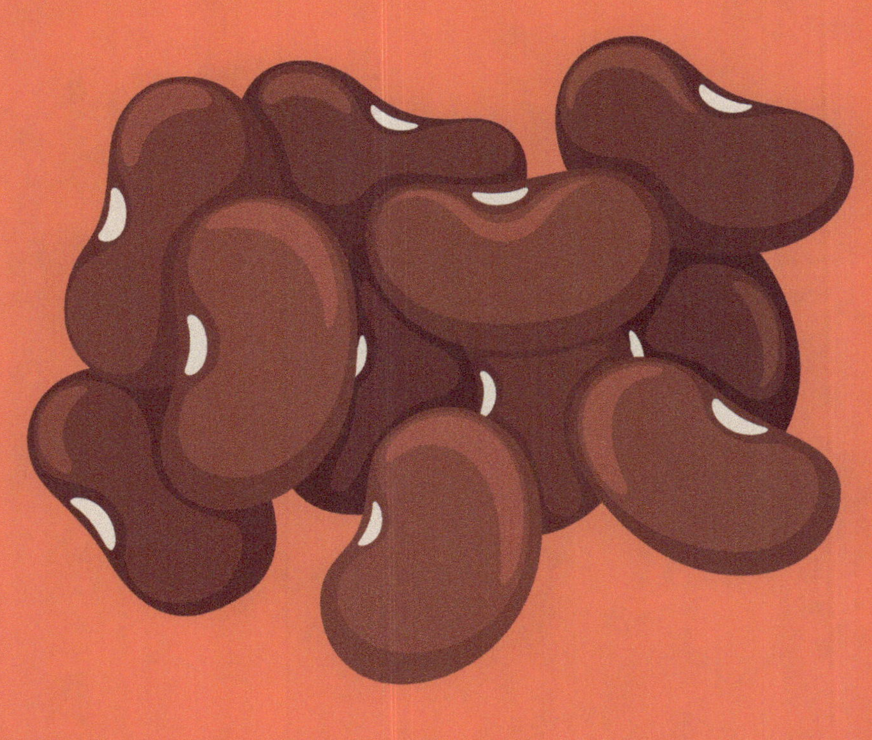

BEANS

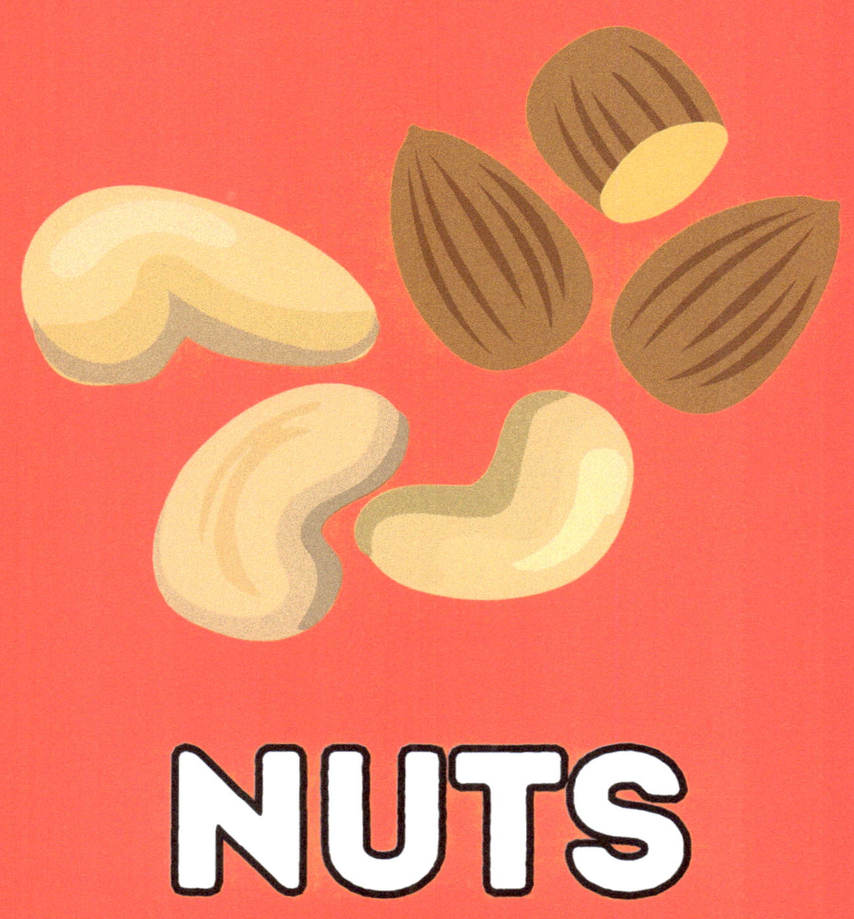

NUTS

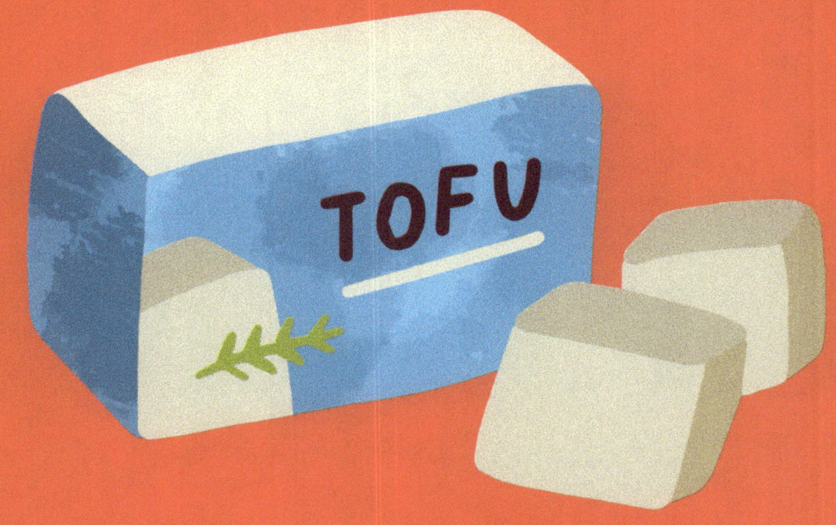

SOY
BASED FOOD

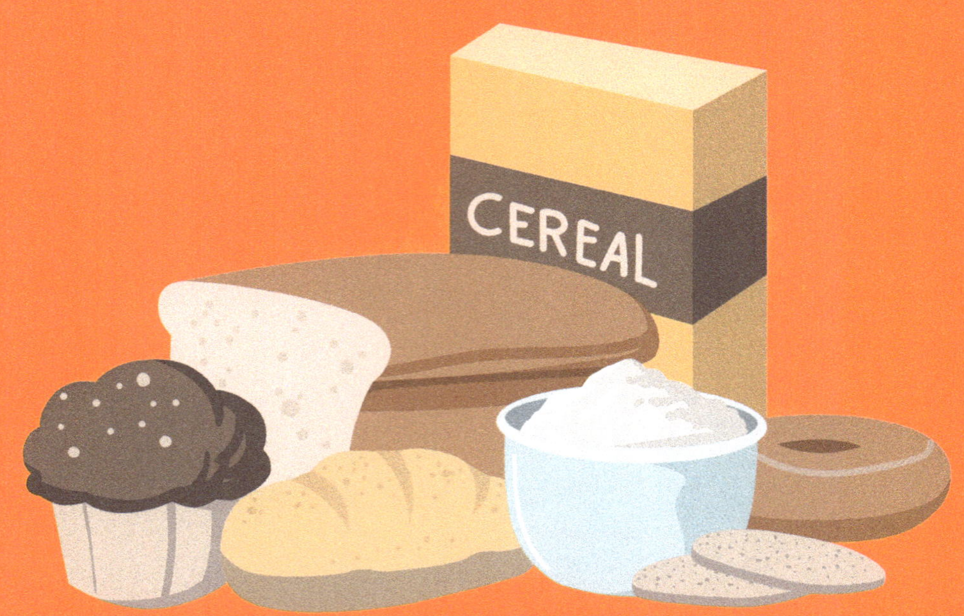

GRAINS

THESE FOODS PROVIDE
US WITH ENERGY
TO RUN, PLAY, AND LEARN!

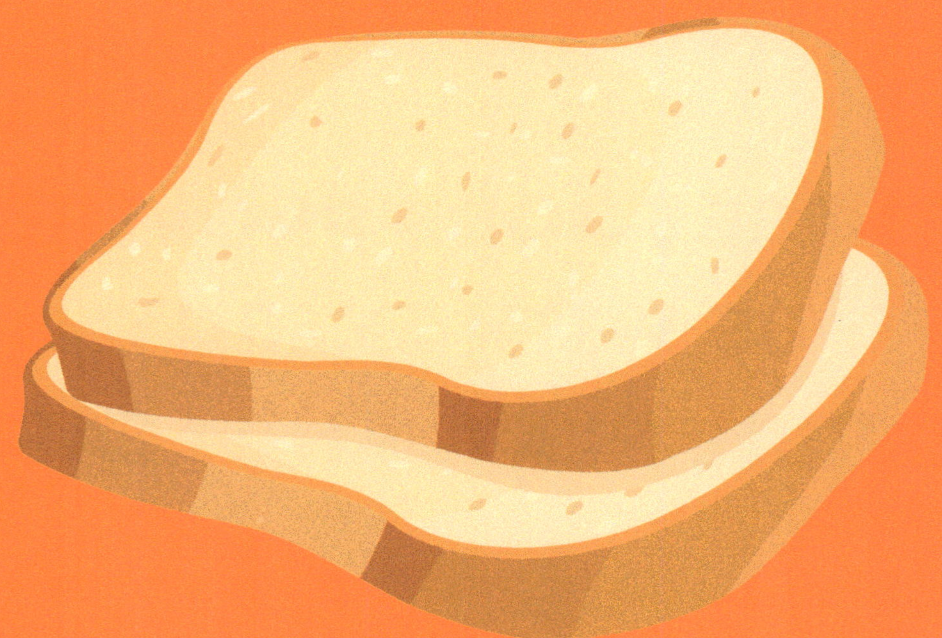

BREAD

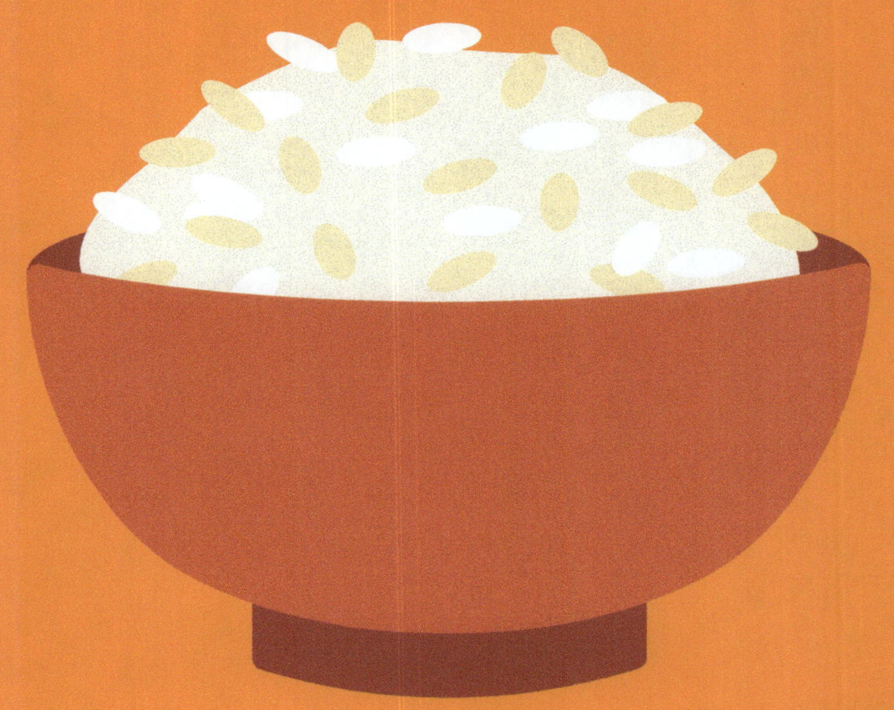

RICE

PASTA

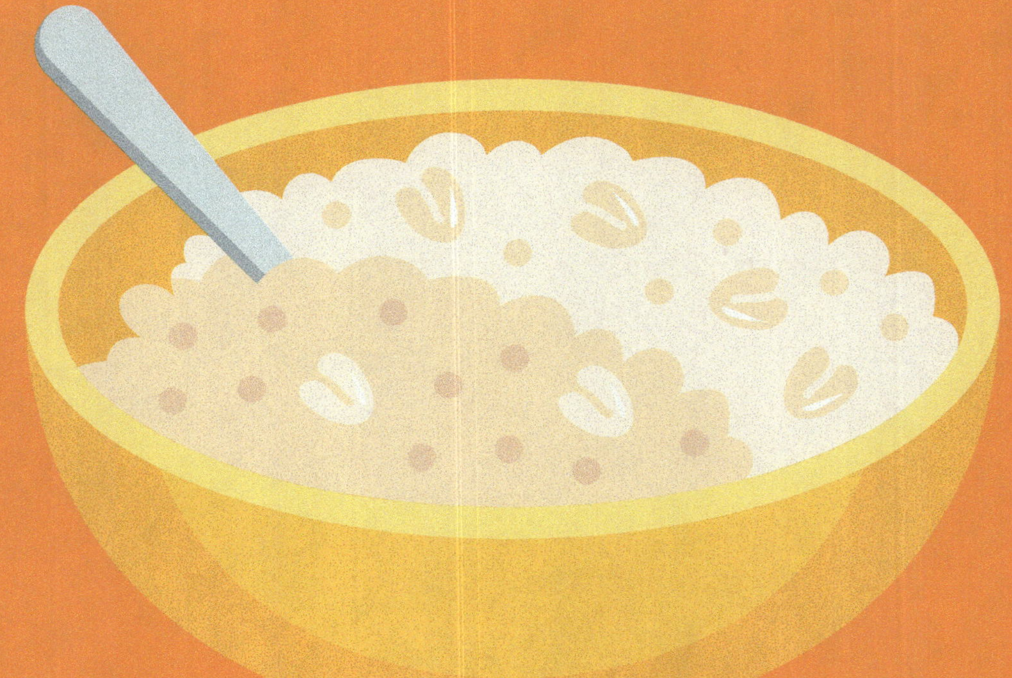

OATS

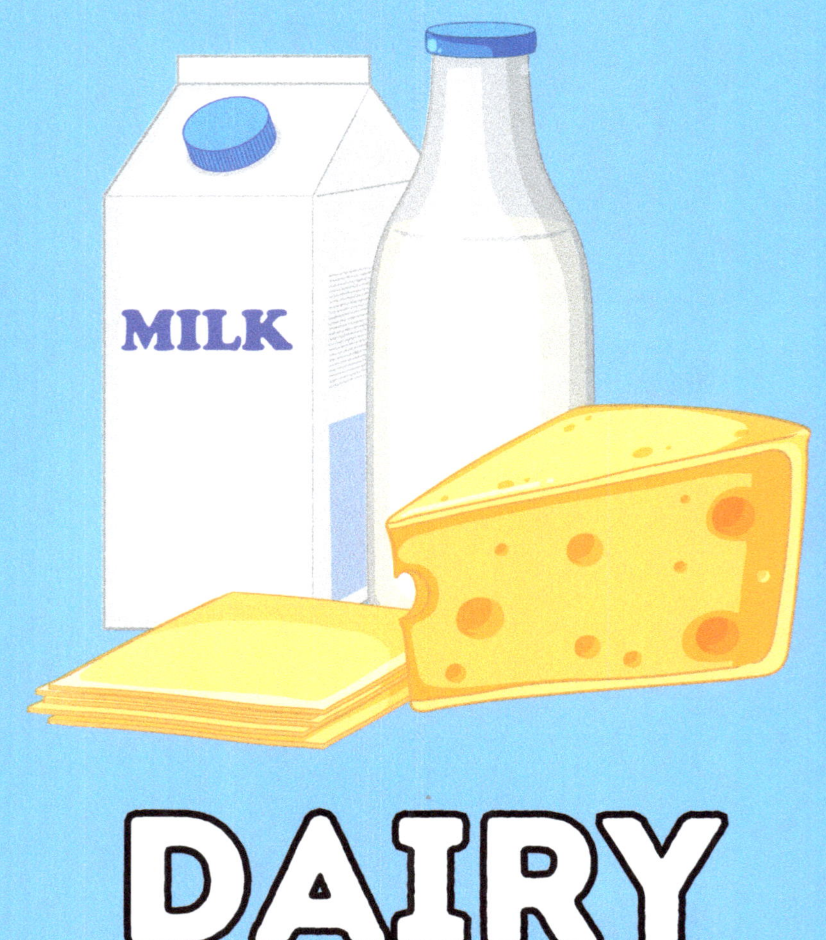

DAIRY

THESE FOODS
GIVE US CALCIUM
THAT MAKES OUR
BONES AND TEETH STURDY.

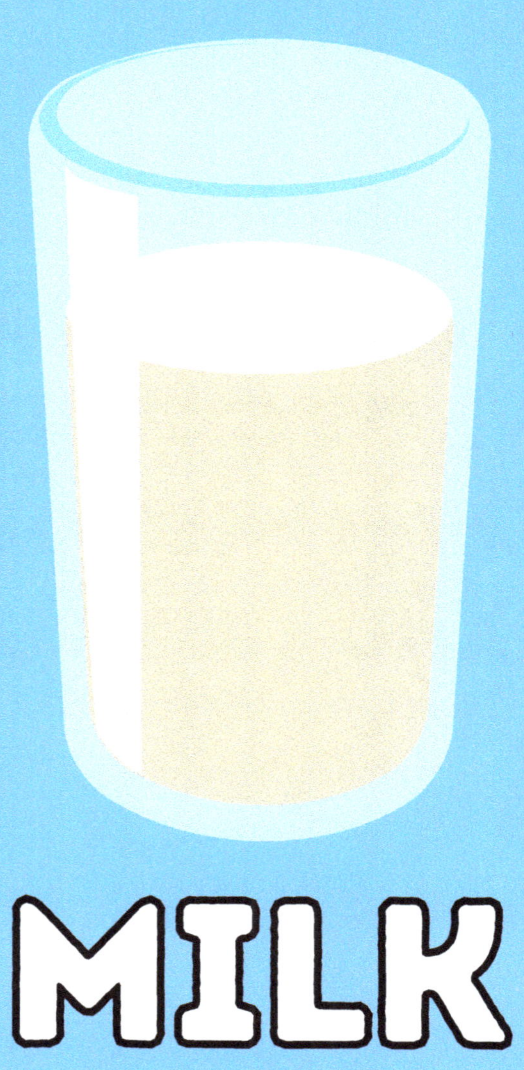

MILK

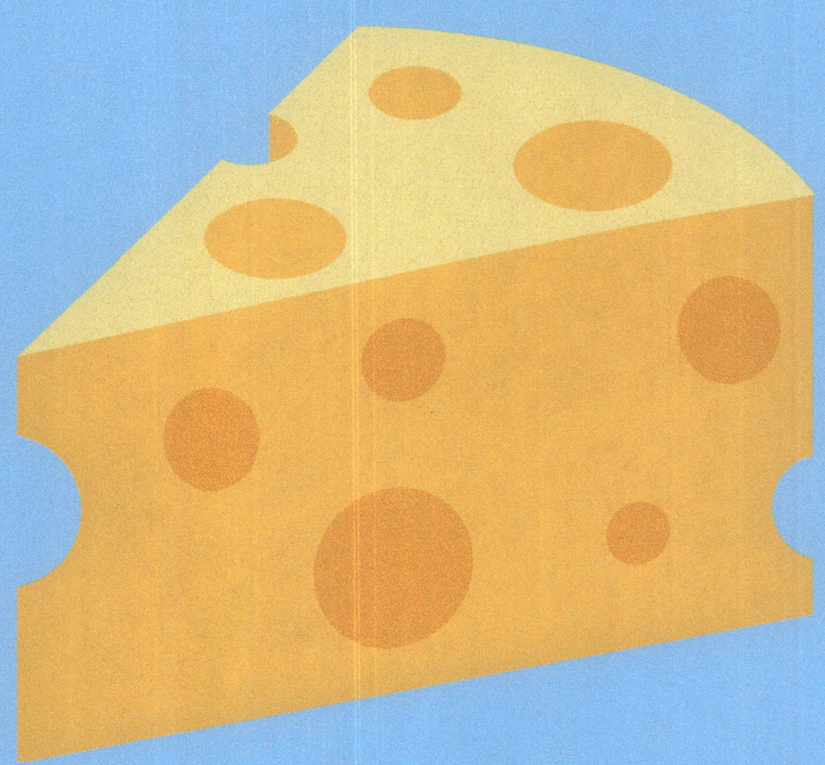

CHEESE

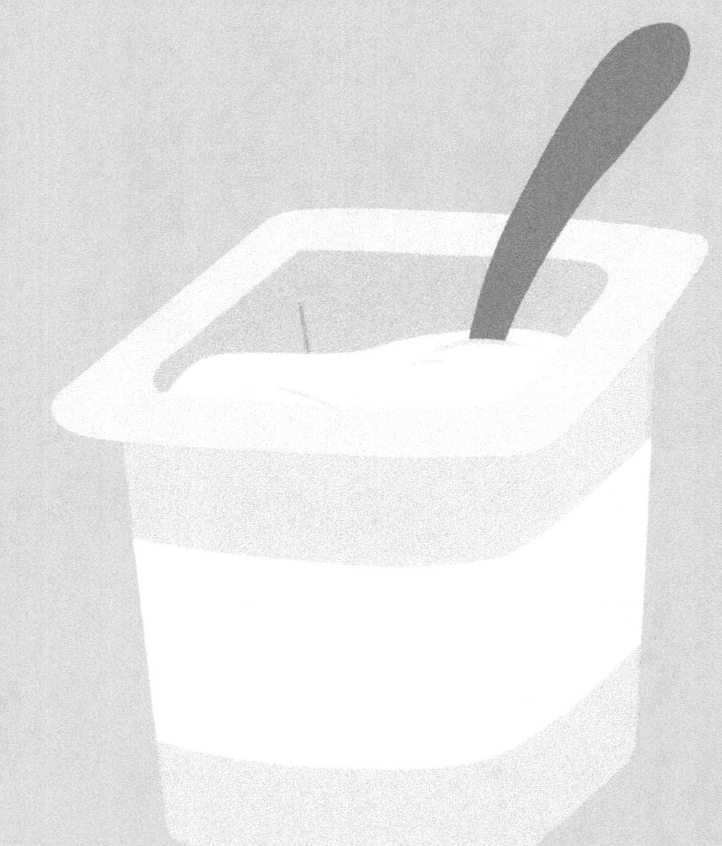

YOGURT

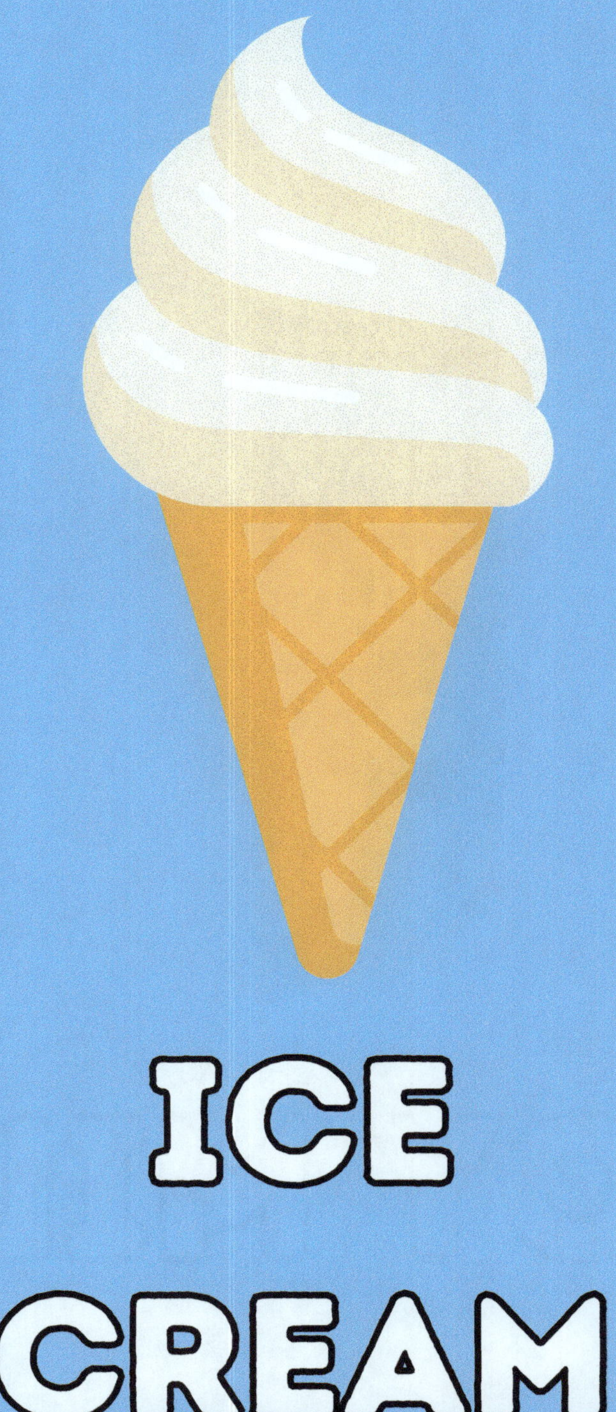

ICE

CREAM

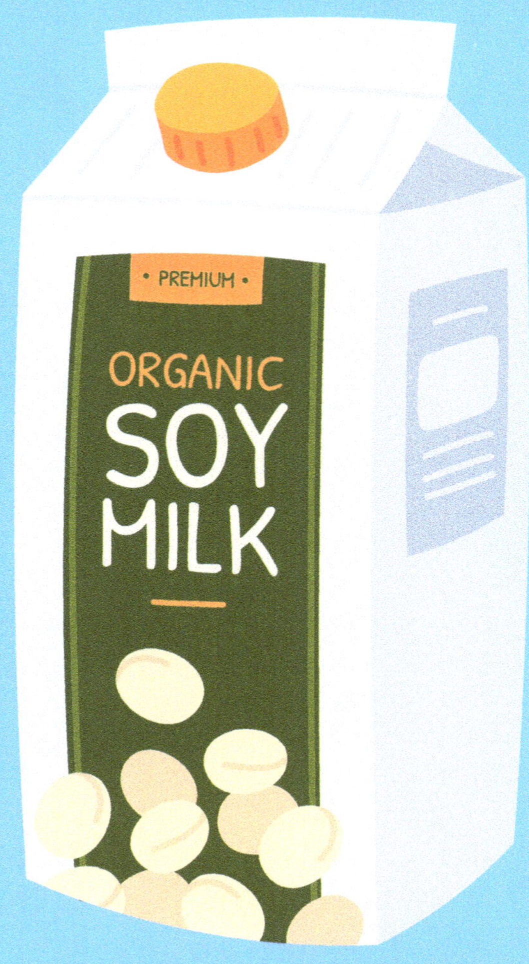

SOY MILK

MAKE YOUR PLATE COLORFUL!

FILL YOUR PLATE EACH MEAL WITH A VARIETY OF COLORFUL FRUITS AND VEGETABLES TO GET A WIDE RANGE OF NUTRIENTS.

BREAKFAST

**SNACK ON
FRUITS AND VEGETABLES
BETWEEN MEALS.**

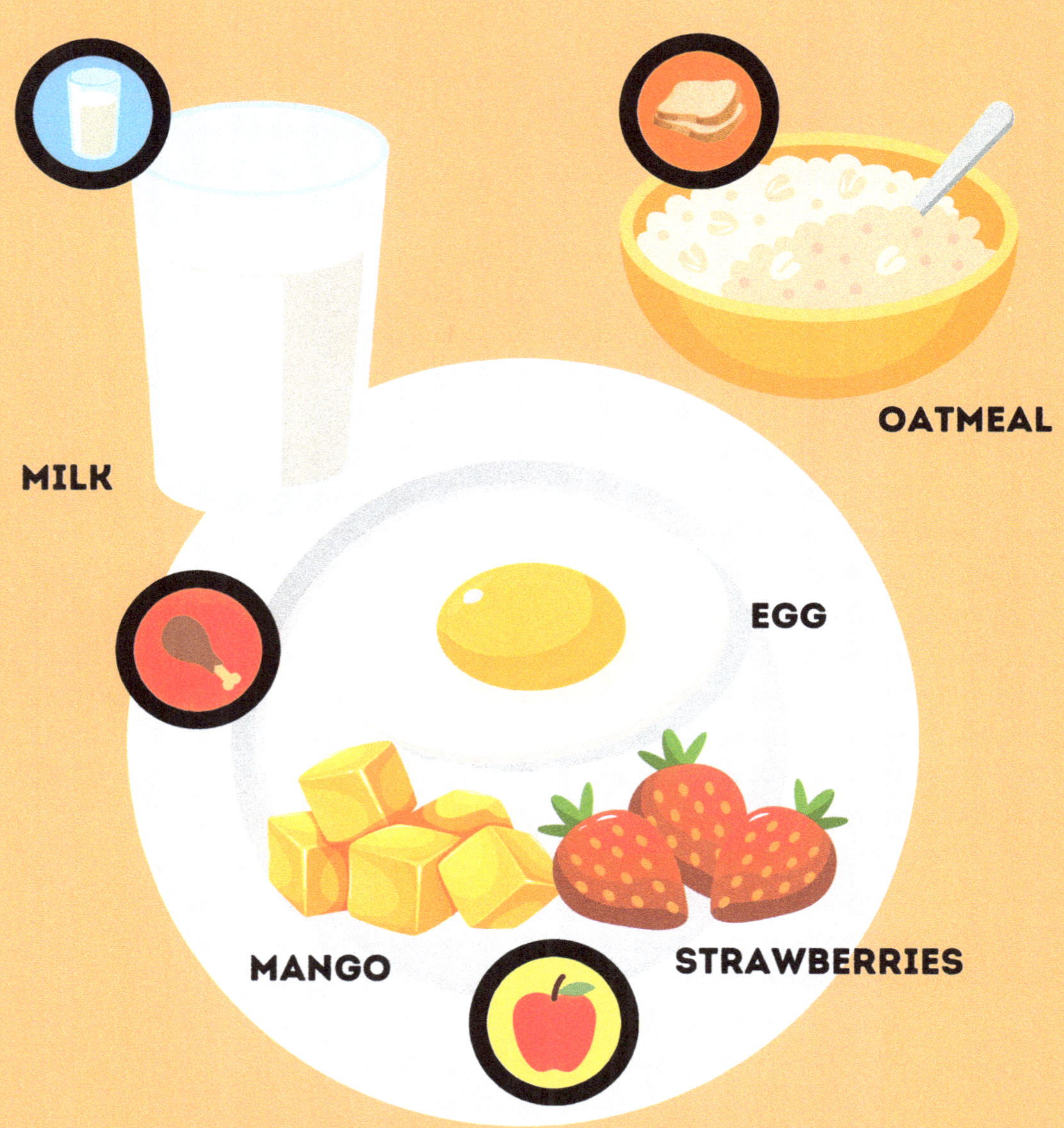

MILK
OATMEAL
EGG
MANGO
STRAWBERRIES

LUNCH

A SANDWICH WITH LEAN MEAT, CRUNCHY VEGGIES AND WHOLE GRAINS WITH A DELICIOUS YOGURT , WILL KEEP YOU FOCUS DURING THE AFTERNOON!

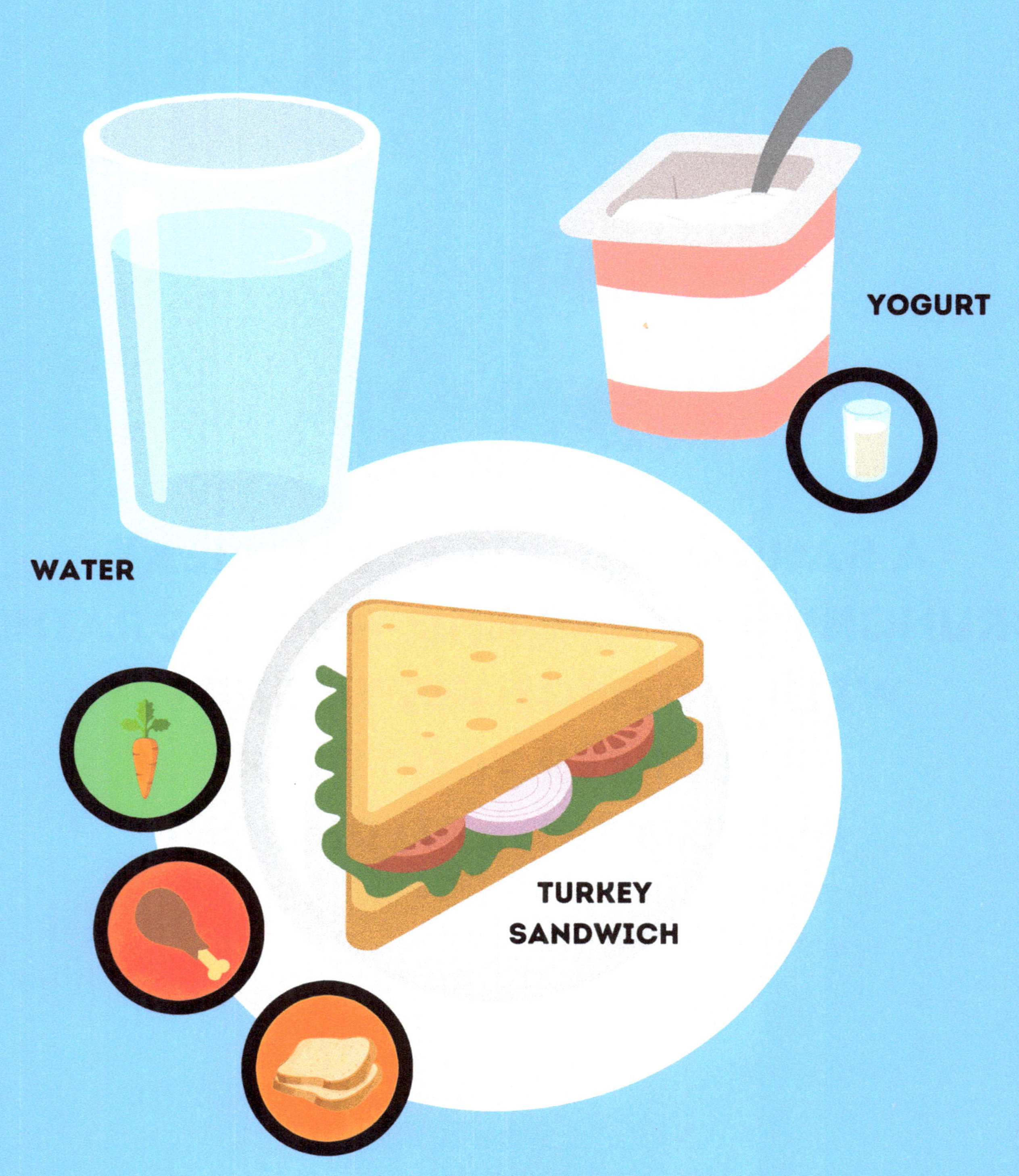
WATER
YOGURT
TURKEY
SANDWICH

SNACK SMART!

**SNACK ON
FRUITS AND VEGETABLES
BETWEEN MEALS.**

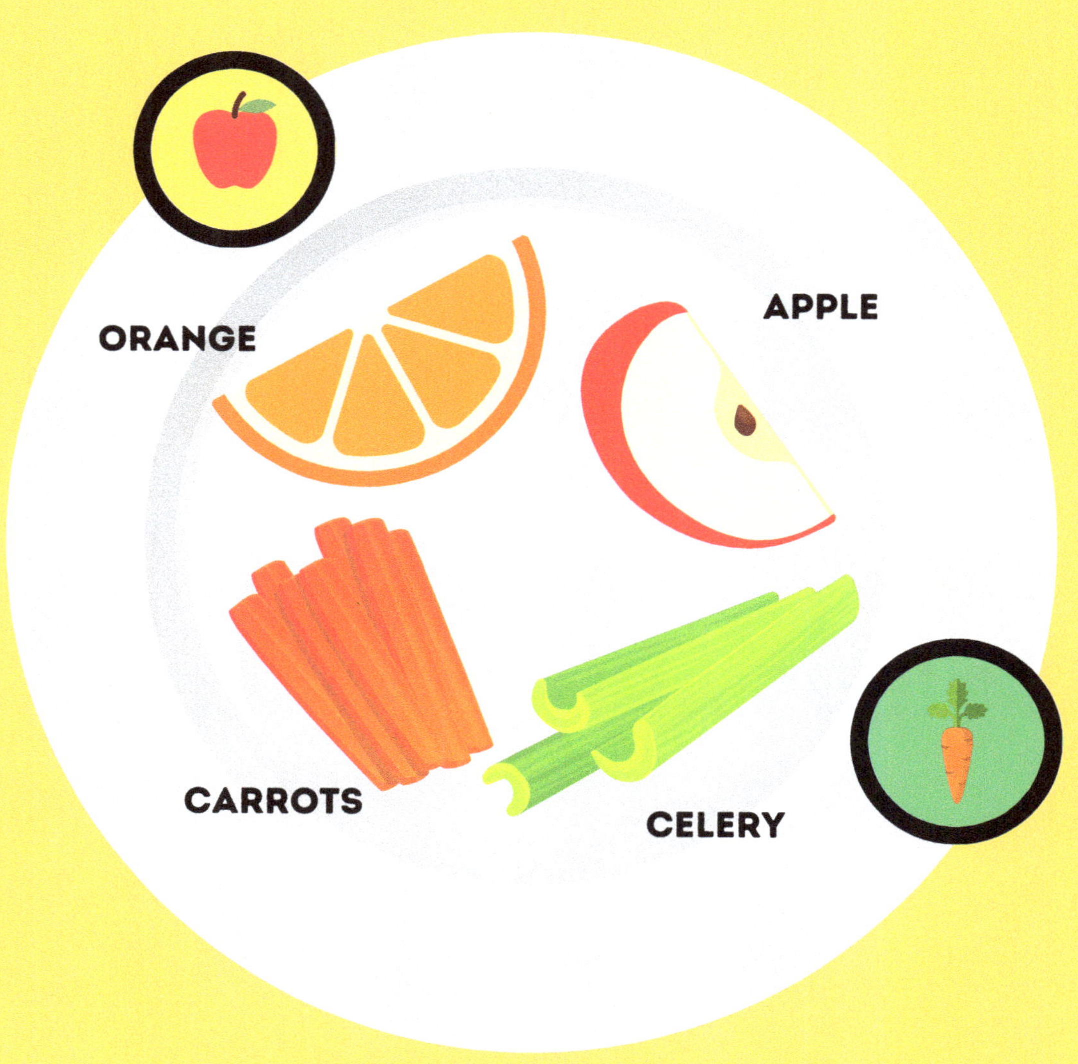

ORANGE
APPLE
CARROTS
CELERY

DINNER

SNACK ON
FRUITS AND VEGETABLES
BETWEEN MEALS.

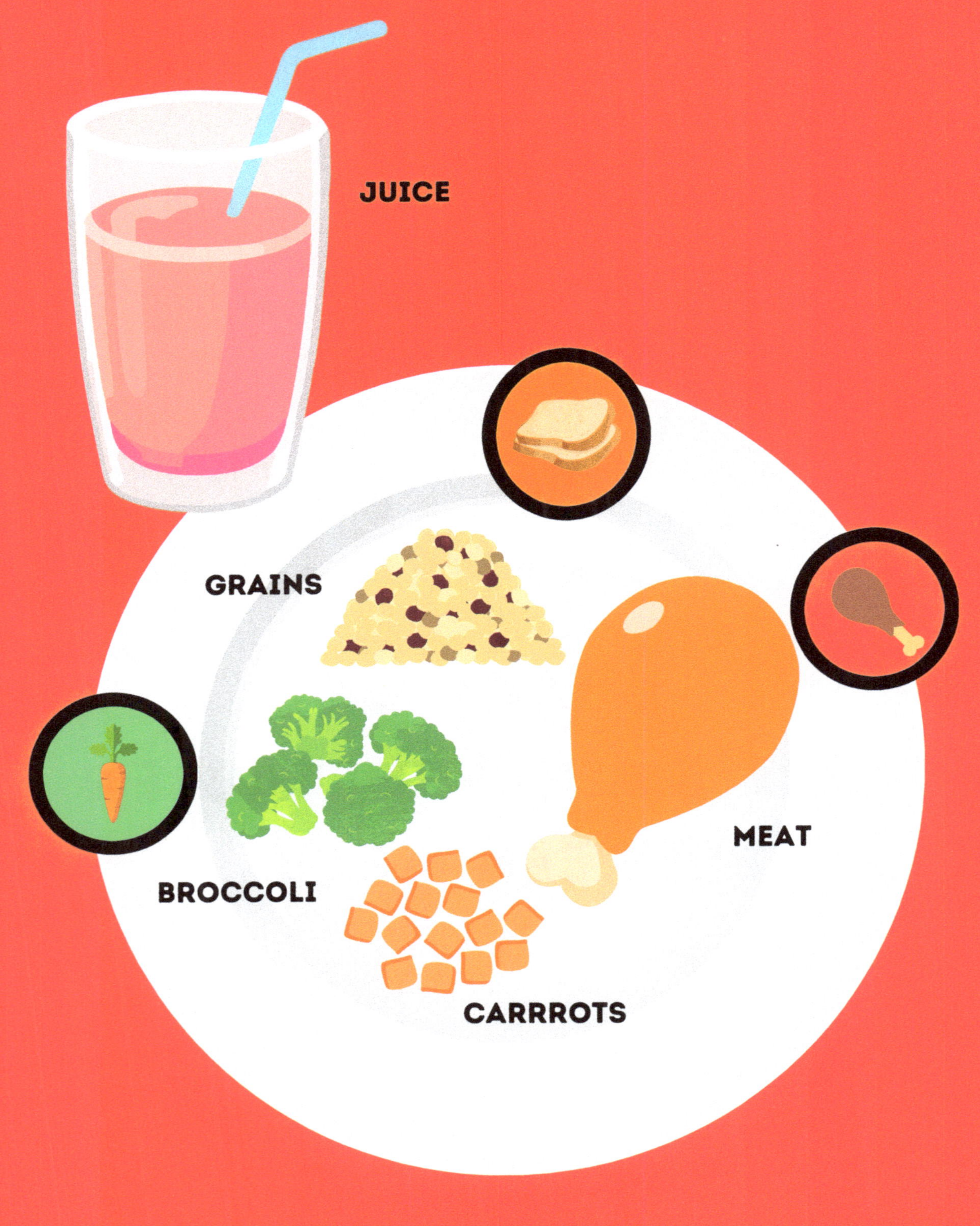

JUICE
GRAINS
BROCCOLI
CARRROTS
MEAT

REMEMBER!

**EATING FROM
ALL THE FOOD GROUPS
HELPS US STAY HEALTHY
AND GIVES US THE ENERGY
TO BE AWESOME EVERY DAY!**

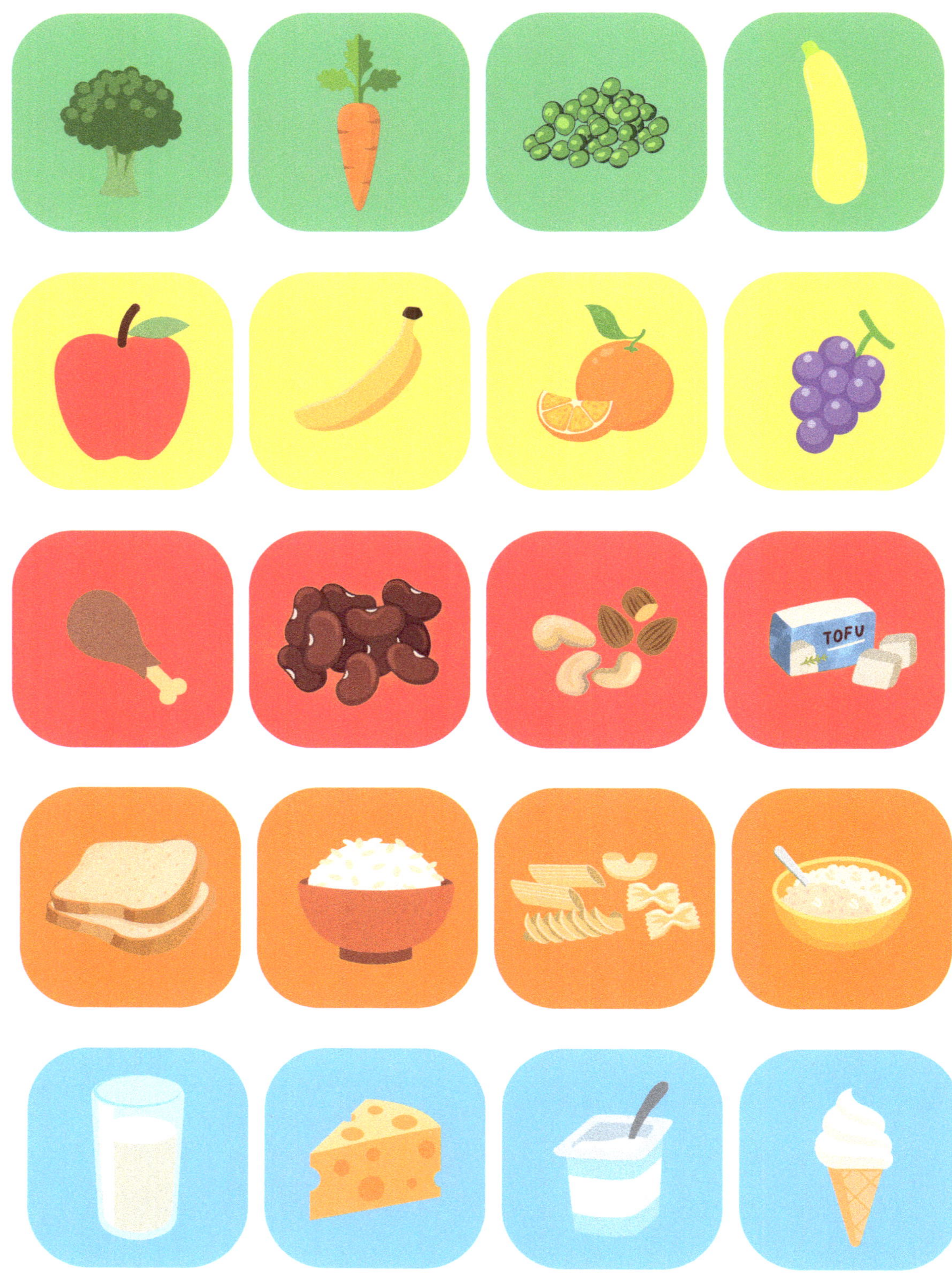